Your Key to Good Health

The Amazing **Endocrine** System

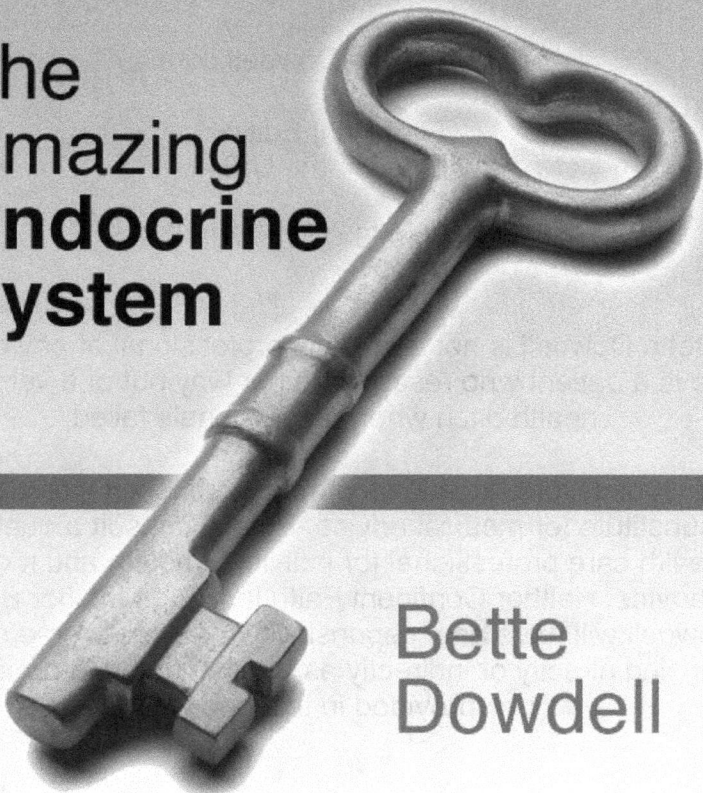

Bette Dowdell

Your Key to Good Health:
The Amazing Endocrine System

published by
Confident Faith Institute LLC
PO Box 11744
Glendale AZ 85318

http://BetteDowdell.com

First Print Edition
Printed in the U.S.A.

ISBN#: 978-0-0717728-9-2

Bette Dowdell is not a medical professional of any sort;
she is a patient who researched her way out of a very deep
health ditch when professionals failed.

Cover by Dairrell Ham, dairrell@gmail.com

Your Key to Good Health: The Amazing Endocrine System

Contents

1. Welcome. 5
2. Introduction. 9
3. How the Whole Thing Works. 11
4. Presenting the Cast. 15
5. The Unknown Hypothalamus. 19
6. Leader of the Endocrine Band: The Pituitary. 23
7. The Metabolism Maestro: The Thyroid. 31
8. The Keep-the-Beat Adrenals. 43
9. The Sugar-Balancing Pancreas. 47
10. The Endangered Gonads. 49
11. Your Protector: The Thymus. 53
12. The Balancing Parathyroids. 55
13. The Mysterious Pineal. 57
14. Leptin: Courtesy of Your Fat. 59
15. Can These Bones Walk?. 61
16. Digestion. 63
17. Symptoms. 65
18. The Problem with Doctors. 69
19. Endocrine Enemies. 73
20. Resources. 74

   Index. 77

Welcome: Prepare to Be Amazed!

If you have health problems, you have endocrine problems. The two always go together, but most of us have no idea what the endocrine system is or what it does. So let's start filling in some blanks.

Quite simply, our endocrine system–thyroid, adrenals, pancreas, thymus, pineal, pituitary, hypothalamus, parathyroids, ovaries and testes, bones and fat–control what happens in our bodies. If they get in trouble, down you go.

But this isn't what you hear–if you hear the word "endocrine" at all. I had to learn how the body works because life presented me with the choice of living brain-dead and bald–or figuring things out.

My endocrine education didn't arrive overnight, either. I spent more than thirty years digging, digging, digging. Now I want to share all those years of learning with you.

We can't find answers until we understand the problem, and we'll never discover ways to prevent or reverse health problems until we learn what the endocrine system does and how to keep it on the straight and narrow.

Allow me to explain my interest in things endocrine.

http://BetteDowdell.com

A month before my first birthday, a drunk driver hit my parent's car, badly injuring my dad and nearly killing my mom. And I torpedoed head first into the car door.

Doctors marveled at my resiliency, announcing I had come through unscathed. But while I looked just fine, I had suffered a concussion, damaging my pituitary gland–as most concussions do.

Doctors continued to insist I was fine for years–as my health slipped away. I finally realized it was up to me.

My mom never recovered from the traumatic brain injury she suffered in the accident and eventually drifted into Parkinson's Disease, a disaster you wouldn't wish on anybody.

Since we shared many of the same symptoms–fatigue, brain fog, etc.–I tried to help her by sharing my discoveries. But she'd demand to know what medical school I had attended and, since I wasn't a doctor, reject what I said.

Parkinson's brings along fear and distrust, so her attitude made sense, kind of. But it meant I couldn't help.

All I could do was double down on my efforts so I didn't end up in the same place she did. And it worked. Staring down Parkinson's Disease focuses the mind wonderfully well.

Through it all, I learned some major truths. First, you can't be healthy unless your endocrine system is healthy. Whether the endocrine system creates the problem, which is likely, or doesn't, it plays a big role.

Second, the endocrine system is a nutrition hog. Without good nutrition, it's a goner. Adding to the problem, most of what we think we know about nutrition is wrong.

http://BetteDowdell.com

Third, nutritional solutions work better than meds. Doctors take one look at my rejuvenated self and tell me if I had really had pituitary problems, I'd be long since dead. Well, I was diagnosed, after extensive testing, by a doctor who was internationally recognized for his diagnostic skills, and experience confirmed that he got it right. Even so, had I not charted my own course, I probably wouldn't have lasted long.

As it is, I'm singing, dancing and living large. And I want the same for you.

Age only means disease if you let it.

This book starts you on the road to better health by introducing you to the endocrine system–which few of us know, let alone understand. You'll get an idea of what the endocrine glands are supposed to do and how to tell if they're in trouble.

The "Resources" chapter describes some solutions I developed through my research and experiences.

Read on.

God is good,
Bette Dowdell

"Bette" has two syllables
"Dowdell" rhymes with "cowbell"

Introduction

Gather round as I tell you about something so important that it controls almost everything that goes on inside your body, but so secret that almost nobody knows about it. Oh, a few may know the name of it, but they couldn't explain it to you–even if you offered them a million dollars.

What is this important, mysterious thing? The endocrine system.

Your endocrine system tells your body how to work–or not. If your brain gets fogged over, think endocrine. If your hair wanders off, think endocrine. If your weight keeps ballooning no matter what you do, think endocrine. If you get an autoimmune disease, think endocrine. Heck, whatever happens, at least give a thought to the endocrine system.

You want amazing? Check out the endocrine system. Not only does the list of activities go on and on, the level of cooperation between endocrine glands goes to the death. If one gland starts to falter, the others try to help. If one gland dies, the others throw themselves on the funeral pyre in an attempt to make things better.

Adding to the merriment, since every endocrine gland maintains a constant conversation, back and forth 24/7, with all the others, in a looped feedback kind of system, they react immediately.

http://BetteDowdell.com

And don't ever decide you can have a problem with only one endocrine gland. One gland may outdo the others in creating a mess, but they're all in there, bailing like crazy.

Plus, all the endocrine glands work in all parts of the body. Receptors for thyroid hormone, for instance, are in the gut, and estrogen receptors are in the brain. Well, who knew?

Endocrine problems are systemwide, and everything affects everything. To use an expression from my old IBM days, a flow chart of what goes on would look like an explosion in a spaghetti factory.

That said, to make any kind of sense, I'm going to write about one gland at time. Just keep a thought in the back of your mind that nothing in the endocrine system acts independently and don't skip a gland or two because you don't think they apply.

I'll write about the hypothalamus, pituitary, thyroid, adrenals, parathyroids, pancreas, pineal, thymus, gonads, leptin, which is not actually a gland, but a real player in the endocrine game, and your bones. Bones? Yup.

One final thought: Whenever you hear the word 'hormone,' you know the topic is the endocrine system–the source of our hormones. And hormones are the gas that keeps the engine running.

How the Whole Thing Works

Everybody has an endocrine system. At least half of them don't work right. And most of that 50% struggle every day–if only trying to locate the bus that hit them.

Must've been a bus. Well, maybe a truck. It had to be something big to flatten us so completely.

We don't know what caused the problem, why it had to pick on us or how to fix it.

Meanwhile, doctors tell us we're 'fine.' We know we're not 'fine,' but we don't know what to do about it.

With this book, I aim to help you understand what your endocrine system does and how it works. Knowing how the pieces fit helps a lot.

Now I recognize that you probably never put understanding the endocrine system on your top-ten list of things to do. But sometimes you just have to dig in and do what you have to do to get where you want to be.

First, let's talk about what the endo part of endocrine means. Our bodies have lots of pipes and plumbing taking things hither and yon, but not the endocrine system, which is pretty much plumbing-free. It has to take a very different approach.

http://BetteDowdell.com

Here's how it goes: Endocrine glands emit hormones into the bloodstream. The hormones drift along until they encounter receptors that chemically fit them, with each hormone have its own specific set of receptors. Having found a fit, the hormone locks into the receptor and gets to work. Nothing happens until the hormone/receptor fit happens.

Unfortunately, chemically similar imposters lurk about, ready to enter or take over the receptor before the hormone can get there. Chaos ensues.

While things seem to be working, our hormones lose the power and the glory to do anything.

For instance, iodine gives your thyroid hormone its oomph; no iodine means no pizzazz. But when fluoride, chlorine and/or bromine (a fire retardant used in bread–for reasons unknown, but probably money) get into your body, they take over the receptors intended for iodine.

With no place to go and nothing to do, iodine gets washed away in your urine.

But when thyroid loses its iodine, you end up with thyroid hormone that doesn't work. It's as if you had no thyroid hormone at all.

Here's the real gotcha: Blood tests can't tell the difference between functional, iodine-enriched hormone and the imposter garbage, so they say you're 'fine.' Bald, brain-fogged and tired to death, but 'fine.' The test said so.

Well, iodine's a wimp, but some hormones get even. If you take phony-baloney estrogen into your body, you put yourself in a world of hurt. Whether it's something you eat, plastic containers, the lining in canned foods, parabens in your lotions and potions, birth control pills, whatever–fake estrogen wreaks

    http://BetteDowdell.com

havoc. You end up awash in estrogen, and things run seriously amok.

You can end up with estrogen dominance. Men grow moobs, lose their libido along with their testosterone and can eventually succumb to prostate cancer. Women say 'good-bye' to their libido, too, and 'hello' to PMS, endometriosis, menopause problems, etc. They also increase their odds of breast cancer. Little boys endure a lifetime of low testosterone. No more John Waynes to take care of business; just Pee Wee Hermans. Little girls experience precocious puberty–and a lifetime of estrogen problems, including fertility issues.

And so it goes.

This book gets you started on understanding 'what happens when' and the consequences–both good and bad–of our actions.

Presenting the Cast

While I discuss each endocrine gland as though it worked separately from all the others, the fact is all of them talk back and forth 24/7 in a looped feedback kind of system. Everybody knows what everybody else is doing. And if one shows signs of trouble, the others jump in to help. They may kill themselves in the effort, but they give it up for the team. Endocrine glands never work–or suffer–alone.

Let's start with something that kind of is and kind of isn't an endocrine gland, the **hypothalamus.** The hypothalamus controls both the nervous system and the endocrine system.

I think you should stand and salute every time you read the word 'hypothalamus.' That would slow things way down, but perhaps you'd end up with an appropriate amount of awe.

Because the hypothalamus is under attack, and it's likely you're participating in your own destruction, mostly by what you eat and drink.

King of the endocrine hill is the **pituitary** gland. A tiny teardrop sort of arrangement, the pituitary hangs from the base of the brain, not too far behind the bridge of the nose.

The pituitary, working with the hypothalamus, tells other endocrine glands when to go and when to stop. The thyroid, for example, never acts on its own, but only when the pituitary tells it to.

http://BetteDowdell.com

Concussions can damage a pituitary. One typical study said 68% of people suffering even a mild concussion had a damaged pituitary.

Adding to that, The Pituitary Networking Association's studies say16.8% of us have pituitary tumors. While these tumors are almost always benign, they can really make a mess of things.

Meanwhile, doctors say pituitary problems are rare and don't check. Given my completely whacked pituitary, this attitude miffs me, but there you are.

Our most well-known endocrine gland is the **thyroid**. It controls metabolism and affects everything else. Most of you know about the hair loss, brain fog, extreme fatigue, etc. that accompany an underperforming thyroid gland, hypothyroidism. Some of you have experienced the living on the edge, hair-on-fire sensation of an overactive thyroid, hyperthyroidism.

You can find your butterfly-shaped thyroid in the front of your neck, near the Adam's apple.

Close by the thyroid lies four similarly named, but unrelated, endocrine glands, the **parathyroids**. These tiny glands control our calcium balance. They get into less trouble than the rest of the gang.

Deep in your brain, in its own little Bat Cave, sits the **pineal** (PIN ee uhl) gland. It produces melatonin to help guide and direct our body's clock–and provide raw material throughout the endo system.

Our **thymus** gland lies behind our breast bone. It's all about our immune system. When they talk about the various t-cells that go to war when disease rampages against us, the 'T' is short for thymus cells. They used to believe the gradual loss of the thymus

http://BetteDowdell.com

was a normal part of life, but now they're learning that loss doesn't have to happen. Exciting research going on.

The two **adrenal** glands perch atop the kidneys in your mid-to-upper back. These babies are a real piece of work, with an uncanny ability to get into trouble. They handle our energy and stress.

If heavy stress goes on and on, the adrenals can conk out. They can also go down trying to help a troubled thyroid gland. And if you try to fix an ailing thyroid gland without first doing something about malfunctioning adrenal glands (which doctors do), it's World War III. Adrenal problems are huge.

The **pancreas**, another big problem maker, is below our stomach, front and center, near the bottom of the rib cage. Just to make things more complicated (and who in the world thought that was necessary?), the pancreas is both an exocrine (with tubing to direct its action) organ that distributes digestive enzymes and an endocrine (emitter/receptor) gland that handles our sugar levels.

The exocrine part gets involved in problems like pancreatitis, a painful enlargement of the pancreas, and pancreatic cancer. The endocrine part can falter into diabetes–too much sugar in the blood–and hypoglycemia–too little sugar in the blood.

The **gonads**, testes and ovaries, finish up the traditional list of endocrine organs. They work with estrogen, progesterone and testosterone. Everybody has all three, but in different proportions. And they're mostly out of whack because of the things we eat, the medicines we take, the things in our food supply that shouldn't be there, and on, and on. If you haven't heard of estrogen dominance yet, you will. It's a huge and growing problem, and it needs more attention.

That used to do it in terms of the endocrine system. For years.

But times, they are a'changing. Endocrine poobahs recently added two new members to the endocrine system: Our **body fat** and our **bones**. They have no glands to call home, but what they do and how they do it (emitter/receptor) make them part of the family.

As I mentioned, the endocrine system constantly engages in a round-robin of conversation. That being the case, can you imagine the stories your blubber is telling on you? Sheesh!

Anyway, our white fat is chock-a-block full of endocrine hormones, chief among them being leptin, which tells us when to stop eating, and ghrelin, which encourages us to chow down. Given a typical diet, they lose their way a lot.

Our bones get included in the endocrine system because their constant activity of renewal involves hormones, what with the osteoblasts, which build new bone cells, and osteoclasts, which cart away dead bone cells.

So those are the players. Now for a closer look.

And a peek at coming endocrine attractions.

The Unknown Hypothalamus

The hypothalamus is kinda, sorta a part of the brain. That is, while it's attached to the base of the brain and referred to as part of the brain, the hypothalamus isn't protected by the blood/brain barrier.

A dinky thing about the size of an almond and the shape of a little, lumpy pancake, it's the tiny king of a vast realm.

And its combination of vulnerability and importance can put us in a world of hurt. Unless we get educated, we'll do bad things to our hypothalamus every day.

So what does the hypothalamus do that's such a big deal? It keeps our bodies in balance (homeostasis in medical terms). It controls body temperature, hunger, thirst, fatigue, anger, sex, emotional attachment, our circadian clock–and on, and on.

How? First, it controls our nervous system through neurotransmitters and neuromodulators–which do exactly what their names sound like: Send signals through the nervous system and modulate those signals so they're not too strong or too weak.

Second, the hypothalamus controls the pituitary gland, which, in turn, controls the entire endocrine system–thyroid, adrenals, pancreas, gonads, pineal, parathyroids, thymus, leptin, ghrelin, etc.

And the hypothalamus links the nervous and the endocrine systems so they work together.

http://BetteDowdell.com

The connection between the hypothalamus and the pituitary is so tight that they have their own little circulatory system to pass their signals and hormones. And talk about constant contact! They talk back and forth every second of your life–balancing, balancing, balancing.

Autoimmune diseases–multiple sclerosis, rheumatoid arthritis, Hashimoto thyroiditis, in fact, all autoimmune diseases–point a strong finger of suspicion at the hypothalamus. Neuropathy–nerve pain–comes from hypothalamus problems. In fact, any and all endocrine disorders can originate from a damaged hypothalamus.

You never want to mess with a major player, and the hypothalamus is a big-time major player.

So why do we give it a world of grief day after day? Because nobody ever mentions the problem.

We're told we shouldn't talk about religion or politics in polite company, and somewhere along the way, talking about the hypothalamus joined the ranks of the hush-hush.

Which means it's my kind of topic. So let's talk.

For one thing, our nutrition-deficient food leaves us malnourished, no matter what the scale says. And malnutrition interferes with what the hypothalamus needs to do.

Then we make things worse by eating something containing monosodium glutatmate. MSG takes a big-time swipe at the hypothalamus. Even pokes holes in it.

Then we eat or drink things containing aspartame, and aspartame dropkicks the hypothalamus.

Aspartame and MSG are hypothalamus killers. No sense beating around the bush, as my mother used to say. These things hate you, hate your body, hate your life. Yes, they're that toxic.

And mixing the two, as we often do with, say, a diet Coke and a bag of Doritos, multiplies the damage many times over.

We're talking major damage. And a damaged hypothalamus announces its predicament in various unhappy ways depending on what else is going on in your body.

There are those who excuse aspartame and MSG as 'natural products.' And it's true that both come from life's basic building blocks, amino acids. Amino acids form proteins, and our bodies use aminos as fuel.

Now this certainly sounds promising. But amino acids come with rules, chief of which is they have to be balanced or have a way to balance themselves.

Aspartate, the source of aspartame, and glutamate, the source of MSG, are not balanced and cannot balance themselves. They do one thing and only one thing: Excite our cells, particularly the brain. Specifically the hypothalamus.

Aspartate and glutamate are excitoxins. They rev up our brain cells to a dangerous, toxic level.

Soy is chock-a-block full of glutamate. And as if taking a whack at the hypothalamus wasn't enough, soy also tromps on the thyroid. Not to mention skyrocketing our estrogen levels.

And when they shoot us up with vaccines, the glutamate in vaccines punches the hypothalamus.

Simply put, aspartate and glutamate torch the hypothalamus. It loses its ability to do all it needs to do, and we go down the tubes.

Here come any number of endocrine problems–including a hit to the immunity-protecting thymus. Here come autoimmune diseases. Here comes peripheral neuropathy. Here comes a world of hurt and woe–and nobody warns us.

Well, consider this your warning. Written in all caps, big, red and blinking. Now you know why disease rates have skyrocketed in the last 40 years.

You need to be considerate, even kind, to your hypothalamus if you want your health to go well.

http://BetteDowdell.com

Leader of the Pack: The Pituitary

The pituitary gland is King of the endocrine hill. The pituitary hangs from the base of the hypothalamus portion of the brain, not too far behind the bridge of the nose, a vulnerable location for such an important actor.

As I said, concussions can cause pituitary damage. That's how I ended up with pituitary problems.

Too many concussions (and nobody knows how many is too many) brings you closer to dementia. And, it seems, to Parkinson's Disease.

Besides concussions, The Pituitary Networking Association's studies say 16.8% of us have pituitary tumors. Most cause no problems, but when they do, it's overwhelming. And they can take years to get diagnosed.

A damaged pituitary means the entire endo system struggles.

If your pituitary doesn't tell your thyroid gland to get it in gear, the thyroid gland does nothing. Your thyroid gland may be able to work, but it doesn't work because it never gets the signal it needs to take action. Since the thyroid gland controls your metabolism, this lack of action is no small matter.

Same with your adrenal glands, from whence you get energy and stress responses. Without a signal from the pituitary, they kick back and do nothing. You're on your own. Again, the adrenals may be ready to rumble, but without a signal, it's as if they failed.

When any endocrine gland doesn't do what it needs to do, all the other glands jump in to help, and it's like the Keystone Kops are in charge.

Here's an example from my own life: When life stressed me, my adrenals didn't kick in to save the day. Minor stresses become major, and major stresses become overwhelming. I had conquered a lot of endocrine problems, but for years, when stress ratcheted up just a little too high, I cried. Which yanked my stress levels a whole lot higher. Do you realize how much power you lose by crying? Nobody wants to blubber in, say, a tax audit, but going in, I knew that could happen.

An aside: I started a tax hearing, wherein the State of Arizona wanted a bunch of money, by reading a statement describing the problem and assuring the male hearing officer that if I began to weep, he should be aware it was not emotional, but physiological, and I would hate it even more than he would.

The statement raised HIS stress level, but a girl's gotta do what a girl's gotta do.

This way, a sudden flood of tears wouldn't undercut my negotiating position as much as if I tried to explain it after the fact. Plus, it guaranteed me his full attention.

He expressed great relief when I made it to the finish line dry-eyed. Me, too. I believed I had found a solution, and surviving the audit dry-eyed confirmed it.

And so it goes. A whacked pituitary causes a lot of grief. Especially since doctors don't help so much.

But I haven't let that stop me, so don't let it stop you, either.

http://BetteDowdell.com

The pituitary gland controls all our hormones, which means the entire endocrine system–pituitary, thyroid, adrenals, pancreas, parathyroids, pineal, thymus, testes and ovaries–and the latest additions, body fat and bones.

As I mentioned, every part of this complex system communicates endlessly–with each other, the pituitary and the hypothalamus. This may be the world's chattiest community. All with a goal of keeping our bodies in balance.

Here's an example of how it goes: The hypothalamus sees that the thyroid gland needs put out a shot of hormone. (Everything happens in intermittent bursts, no steady flows.) The hypothalamus then sends a shot of TRH to the pituitary, telling it to send a shot of TSH to the thyroid. When the TSH hits, the thyroid gives off thyroid hormone–at which point the hypothalamus says "enough already" and sends a stop message to the pituitary, which sends a stop message to the thyroid. How often this relay happens depends on how much thyroid hormone you need for your activities.

Keep in mind, the thyroid is also talking–to the pituitary and other parts of the endocrine system while this goes on. And getting input from all the others, too. Our endocrine system is one amazing piece of work.

You'll have difficulty finding a doctor willing to investigate pituitary problems. Amazingly, I've found endocrinologists to be the worst! Keep searching; they're out there–somewhere.

The sections of the pituitary

The pituitary has three known sections: Anterior, intermediate and posterior lobes, each with different functions.

Opinions vary on the functions of the **intermediate lobe**. This section of the pituitary produces a hormone, melanocyte, which affects skin pigmentation. Some say it causes freckles, moles, etc. Some say it loses function early on in life.

Recent research, though, reveals it plays a major, previously unsuspected role of signaling the posterior and anterior lobes when to take action or not take action, so it seems to be in charge. Stay tuned.

The **posterior lobe** holds the **oxytocin** and **vasopressin** created by the hypothalamus, emitting them as needed. If you've heard of oxytocin at all, it's probably as the hormone that starts and paces labor–which doesn't begin to tell the story.

Oxytocin provides the glue that keeps personal relationships together–romantic relations, friends, siblings, kids, all relationships. It helps regulate our cardiovascular system, improves our memory, gives us confidence and plays a huge role in all parts of the endocrine system.

Interestingly, promiscuity diminishes oxytocin levels and makes it harder to maintain any relationship. And low oxytocin whacks our health for good measure .

Vasopressin, also called antidiuretic hormone (ADH), is very similar chemically to oxytocin, and shares some of its functions, but vasopressin works mainly to regulate the blood's water, glucose and salt levels through anti-diuretic action–when and if we need it.

The **anterior lobe** controls a large part of what the pituitary does. It sends out TSH to get the thyroid going, ACTH for the adrenals, luteinizing and follicle stimulating hormones for the gonads, etc. We get our growth hormone here, too. We're talking busy, busy, busy.

If the anterior lobe fails, the other endocrine glands don't get their stop-and-go signals. It's possible for only one or all parts of the anterior lobe to fail, but a failure of two or three parts (like, say, those affecting the thyroid and adrenals) is more common.

They say failure of all three pituitary lobes (panhypopituitarism), which is my problem, rarely happens. And if it does happen, they add, there's no way to make things better. I'm glad I didn't believe them.

They test for pituitary tumors with an MRI. Beyond that, they check individual endocrine glands, assuming the problem's there, not in the pituitary.

But low thyroid may not be a thyroid problem; it could be a pituitary or hypothalamus problem. Maybe the pituitary can't respond to the hypothalamus. Or maybe the hypothalamus isn't talking. And so on.

They could test the hypothalamus to see if it's sending out hormones for the pituitary to act on, but they don't. And they could test the pituitary hormones, but these tests only seem to happen in research settings. I can't begin to guess why that is, but I'm guessing there's a dollar sign in there somewhere.

Symptoms of pituitary problems mimic those of other endocrine glands, but a few symptoms can raise suspicions. A lack of growth hormone shows up noticeably when children fail to grow; the same lack in adults means faster aging, but who knows what's normal in something you only do once? You'll need more specific evidence than just feeling old to have a chance at getting tested.

Loss of underarm and pubic hair suggest pituitary problems. As do joint stiffness, constant hoarseness, epic mood swings and loss of memory. Since each of these symptoms can arise from other health issues, you'll probably need a cluster of them to stir a doctor's interest.

http://BetteDowdell.com

Let's face it. Telling the doctor you want your pituitary tested because your armpits are bald won't get you very far. Especially since it may well come as news to the doctor that bald armpits and pituitary problems are related.

Concussions

We need to talk about the impact a concussion can have on the pituitary.

Doctors don't check for it. Articles in popular magazines don't talk about it. It's just not on our radar, but it should be.

Even a mild concussion can cause a lifetime of hurt. In a concussion, our brains bang around against our skulls, and the poor little pituitary takes a real beating.

The whole endocrine system suffers when the King is halfway off the throne and not really ruling the kingdom. Problems may arise quickly, or they may show up years later, but sooner or later, things start falling apart–the thyroid, adrenals, pancreas, etc.

You look fine. People think you are fine. But you aren't fine.

I tell you all of this because to fix a problem, you have to know what it is. Perhaps you've been wondering why you feel like death struck by a brick.

Doctors don't take concussions seriously most of the time, and they may not even tell you they suspect you have one. Be sure to ask.

Why not just let the doctor handle it? Because full recovery requires a big dose of do-it-yourself action.

Now starteth the sermon: Don't listen to anybody who says you have no reason to hope for better days if you don't heal quickly. I disagree. Decide not to have anything to do with hopelessness.

Passivity loses most of its battles. So don't even think for an instant that you should give up and spend the rest of your days doing beached whale impressions. Not ever. Get your "OH, YEAH!" attitude on and take care of business.

The Metabolism Maestro:
Your Thyroid

Our most well-known endocrine gland is the thyroid. Historically, 20% of the population had thyroid problems. Nowadays, it's up to 50%. That's a whole lot of misery.

The thyroid, a butterfly-shaped gland located by your Adam's apple, affects everything that goes on in your body. When the thyroid ain't happy, ain't nothing happy.

You probably know about the weight problems, hair loss, brain fog, depression, extreme fatigue, etc. that accompany an underperforming thyroid gland. Some of you have experienced the heart palpitations, eye problems and anxiety of an overactive thyroid.

Hyper and hypo share some of the same symptoms, but hypo people generally feel like a pile of mush that doesn't want to move while hyper people feel tired, but wired.

Whether hypo or hyper, you never lack for a boatload of symptoms. One reference book lists slightly more than 300 symptoms for hypothyroidism alone. Is it any wonder, then, that doctors don't want to hear about them?

Doctors prefer blood tests to symptoms. And who could complain–if the tests worked. Which they don't.

http://BetteDowdell.com

The so-called gold standard of thyroid tests–the TSH–came to us based on a vote of endocrinologists, not science. They keep moving the goal posts to make things come out right, but that doggone test won't cooperate. Never mind. Full speed ahead. And millions of people drag through life because doctors won't listen to their symptoms, and they 'fail' the TSH test.

Research shows that one form of hypothyroidism, inherited from mothers, never passes the TSH–or any other test. Type 2 hypothyroidism, as it's called, is all about symptoms. The tests have nothing to do with anything, so those patients, perhaps a majority of hypothyroid people, rarely get treated.

Thyroid tests throw a major curve into treatment. Tests can give normal results even when you're in a heap on the floor verging on comatose or, alternately, leaping tall buildings in a single bound. Thyroid treatment can't be about routine tests; it has to be about symptoms.

Untreated or undertreated low thyroid function leads to heart disease, fibromyalgia, adrenal failure, auto-immune diseases, and on, and on. All added, of course, to the pile of symptoms you started with.

Well, it's all pretty daunting. And while we can't ask for a redeal on the hand life gave us, we can play the hand wisely. Look for a doctor willing to treat symptoms. Avoid bad things that drag you down. Adopt the diet, vitamins and minerals that build you up.

I'm here to help.

A Look at Thyroid Tests

Thyroid tests come from theory, not hard science. Theories can eventually be proved, of course, but until that happens, you don't want to bet your health on a theory.

http://BetteDowdell.com

And thyroid tests are still theory, not proven fact.

For instance, the TSH test. Logic says if our pituitary gland has to keep nagging the thyroid to work harder, it must mean the thyroid isn't keeping up. Is that really how it works? Perhaps. Kinda seems so. But we have no science to confirm it.

Here's the theory:

When the thyroid needs to run faster, the hypothalamus signals the pituitary, the pituitary sends a shot of thyroid-stimulating hormone to the thyroid, and the thyroid gets it in gear.

When the thyroid needs to slow down, the hypothalamus sends a slow-down signal, the pituitary sends a shot of thyroid-inhibiting hormone to the thyroid, and the thyroid stops pumping out hormone.

This accelerator/brake action goes on all day, every day. Never stops.

The theory concludes, then, that when the thyroid is running too slowly, the pituitary keeps shooting out TSH, and your TSH blood levels rise.

And since theory says the pituitary hoards TSH when the thyroid's off to the races, a low TSH means your pituitary's laying back because your thyroid's running amok and won't stop.

Well, that's the theory. And the basis for the TSH test.

We have some problems here. First, the TSH tests what's happening in the blood, not in the tissues where the action happens.

Second, as a result of concussions and tumors, not everybody's pituitary works; they could test, but they don't.

Third, in the case of inherited thyroid problems, the whole test thing falls apart.

Fourth, they don't test for thyroid inhibiting hormone, the direct sign of a pituitary trying to slow down a raging thyroid.

Fifth, we have no science to prove the TSH test provides accurate information and a lot of anecdotal evidence that says it doesn't.

Sixth, if we take desiccated thyroid, the medication that actually works, our TSH will always be low, signifying nothing.

And then there's the problem of what constitutes a normal TSH level. TSH test ranges have always been a moving target as they tried to make results fit the facts. And now they're thinking the test doesn't work. But they still use it! And how many people crawl through life because of that infernal test?

Why do they keep using it? A blood test lends the appearance of science–and it's certainly easier than listening to a patient's symptoms and figuring out how to make them go away. Which is really hard to do in a ten-minute office visit.

How about the rest of the thyroid tests?

• T4 test et al: Natural thyroid hormone has five parts, T1, T2, T3, T4 and calcitonin. T1 is the amino acid tyrosine with one iodine molecule. T2 is tyrosine with two iodine molecules. And so on. Calcitonin works with the bones and the parathyroid glands.

T4 does very little beyond acting as a storage depot. T3 has the reputation of doing all the heavy lifting. Recent research,

http://BetteDowdell.com

however, says T2 actually does some of what T3 gets credit for. And very recent research suggests T1 is in there pitching, too.

Since medicine believes T1 and T2 do nothing, they don't get tested. Neither does calcitonin.

When you get a thyroid test, besides the TSH, you'll get some combination of the five main tests: T4, T3, Free T4, Free T3 and antibodies.

The T4 and T3 tests don't measure anything that means anything, so they're not used much anymore.

The free T4 and free T3 tests measure the T4/T3 left over in our blood after the tissues are finished using what they need. So they're indirect tests, and, again, test the blood, not the tissues. But doctors like them because it means they don't have to listen to symptoms and deal with the fact that one-size-fits-all medicine doesn't work.

A test for antibodies checks for autoimmune thyroid disease, Graves for hyperthyroidism, Hashimoto's for hypothyroidism. In autoimmune disease, the body wages war on itself, in this case, your thyroid. Your symptoms hop around all over the place, putting you in a world of misery.

And antibody tests don't always tell the story either. If your overall health's in the dumpster, you may be too unhealthy to create antibodies . Eliminating the things that do you in and adding the nutrition that builds you up will make you feel a world better, Then, the healthier-you will create antibodies–just when you thought you had it licked!

Plus antibodies from food sensitivities look like thyroid antibodies–at least to the test. So, which are they? Good question.

http://BetteDowdell.com

Research on antibody tests contradicts the tar out of itself. It's hard to imagine the antibody tests works any better than the rest of the tests.

Once the tests tell their tale, doctors decide how much medicine to give. Since the advent of thyroid blood tests, the average dose of the thyroid medicine given to hypothyroid patients is half of what doctors prescribed when they treated symptoms. So even if we're treated, we're still in a mess.

To add to the mess, doctors prescribe the useless Synthroid or a generic equivalent.

Synthroid and its ugly generic cousins don't work for the vast, vast majority of people, but they make the blood tests (T3, T4, etc.) look like perfection in action. You may be in a heap on the floor gasping for air, but you're fine; the tests say so.

You can only look on in dismayed astonishment as your doctor waves the test result 'evidence' around and declares victory.

Never mind that untreated/under treated hypothyroidism causes the entire endocrine system–the wheel in the middle of the wheel in how our bodies work–to go whacko. Never mind, as well, that it causes heart disease. And a whole list of other health disasters.

In fact, never mind anything, The unscientific, unreliable test has spoken.

Doctors celebrate "evidence-based medicine." Well, the evidence is in, and all the thyroid blood tests get a failing grade. As for Synthroid, is there such a thing as an F-?

If you can, find a doctor who treats patients, not tests.

Thyroid Meds

Hypothyroid: Synthroid, the blood tests' evil twin, came out in the 1960s about the same time as the thyroid blood tests. (Any way you look at it, that was a bad decade.)

First problem: Synthroid stands for synthetic thyroid. Our bodies don't like synthetics unless they're an exact copy of the real thing, which Synthroid isn't.

Second problem: Natural thyroid hormone contains five parts: T4, T3, T2, T1 and calcitonin. Besides being a cheap synthetic, Synthroid contains only T4.

The theory behind Synthroid (again there's no science) says T4, the slow-acting, storage part of thyroid hormone will convert to T3, the active form—which is what we need, as we need it.

Well, not so fast, Chester. Conversion depends on a lot of things. First off, the body doesn't usually recognize the synthetic T4 meds, so how would it know what to convert them to? And some people can't get the job done because their bodies don't know the trick. Additionally, low cholesterol, so praised by doctors, prevents conversion. Not to mention the fact that 95% of us lack the minerals required for the T4/T3 conversion. And I could go on. We can't depend on any conversion.

Without the conversion, of course, we never get any active thyroid hormone, and we feel like death warmed over, but, again, the blood tests say we're fine. No matter how we feel, we're fine.

To get a complete thyroid medication, ask for dessicated thyroid such as Armour, or one of it's generic equivalents. Armour has more than 150 years of excellent history, while Synthroid has a spotty history—and only about fifty years worth at that.

But since Big Pharma money took over medical schools in the 1960s, doctors have been taught to view Armour as the enemy.

http://BetteDowdell.com

Some state medical boards join the anti-patient battle. The FDA handmaidens join in the fray.

As do others. Some HMOs ban Armour. Military doctors can't prescribe it. Medicare doesn't approve. Even without those limits, doctors may not want to prescribe it. Being human, they want other doctors to esteem them, which nobody would if the word got out they were prescribing Armour.

The United Kingdom won't allow natural thyroid to be used by anybody. Other countries may be moving in that direction.

Do you get the idea medicine and politicians don't give a hoot about your health?

Hyperthyroid: Some doctors give you medicine to tame the beast; if one of the meds doesn't work, you have the option of switching to another–and another. Read before you take any of the meds. Solid research is sounding alarm bells.

Other doctors insist on removal of your thyroid gland, either surgically or by radiation–which leaves you hypothyroid. Some do a partial thyroidectomy in hopes of striking a happy balance.

Sacrificing your thyroid to the knife may, unfortunately, include whacking the tiny parathyroids. You end up not only with thyroid problems, but with rampant osteoporosis that nobody knows how to fix.

The problem is you're so beset by symptoms, you're pretty much willing to do whatever you're told.

But did you know that iodine/iodide (Iodoral) was used to fix hyperthyroidism from 1811 to the 1960s when a doctor at the National Institutes of Health took exception to it? (This happened about the same time medicine came up with the TSH test and

Synthroid and took over the medical schools. Some might see a coincidence there.)

Bottom line, neither hypo or hyper get good medical care. Not even reasonable medical care, in fact. You have to engage in the process. Trust yourself–about the treatment, about changing doctors, everything. You're the one who knows how you feel.

Meanwhile, help yourself with a solid vitamin/mineral program and a diet that supports health. Learn how the endocrine system works and cooperate with what needs to happen.

Two traps to avoid
High cholesterol levels accompany thyroid problems. Now, when your thyroid's in trouble, your cholesterol level may be interesting information, but it's not important information.

However, doctors know only one response: Prescribe a statin drug. You do not want to join that party.

Statins cause an avalanche of side effects while curing nothing. Besides, while high cholesterol is safe, even beneficial because once you reach the big 5-0, low cholesterol can kill you. Meanwhile, your thyroid desperately needs cholesterol to function–as does your brain.

Just say "no" to statin drugs.

2. Low thyroid and insufficient stomach acid go together. Without adequate stomach acid, you can't digest the proteins your body badly needs. Adding to the fun, the undigested proteins throw your gut into fits.

Since low stomach acid has the same symptoms as high stomach acid–heartburn, GERD, etc.–and doctors have medicine to "fix" high stomach acid, but nothing for low stomach acid–here cometh a prescription guaranteed to make things worse.

Antacids, whether prescription or over-the-counter, may briefly relieve symptoms, but you're digging a big hole for yourself.

How To Help Your Thyroid
• Don't eat bread, cookies, cakes, etc–at least, not any you buy. And not because of weight. Commercial bakeries started using bromine as a dough conditioner in the 1980s, and bromine means death to the thyroid.

• Eat plenty of protein, including red meat with good saturated fat at least every other day. At least. Our thyroid glands, as part of the endocrine system, thrive on protein and fat. They live for them. They can't make it without them. And red meat has micronutrients we need and can't get anywhere else.

But make it grass-fed beef so you get good fat while avoiding the antibiotics and hormones they feed cows raised on factory farms.

• Avoid high fructose corn syrup. Consider it poison–which it is–and never let it near your lips. Every endocrine gland you own will thank you–not to mention your liver, gall bladder, kidneys, and so on. Probably even your toenails since they'll have an easier time off fighting fungal infections.

• And for pity's sake, I'm begging you, don't eat soy. Or drink soy. Or put soy lotions on your body. Just don't have anything to do with soy.

Besides depressing thyroid function, soy messes with the entire endocrine system, especially estrogen, testosterone and progesterone. Do you really want to do a number on your reproductive system?

Eliminating soy means eliminating 60% of processed foods, which includes fast food, meals at most chain restaurants and any meal that comes out of a box.

• Take quality vitamins and minerals to give your body the ammunition it needs to fight the good fight. Food alone can't do everything that needs doing, so you have to supplement. And you have to supplement intelligently. Picking up any old thing in the grocery store is probably better than nothing, but not wonderful.

The Keep-The-Beat Adrenals

We have two **adrenal** glands, each perched atop a kidney. With your spine dividing your back in two, you can locate a kidney in the middle of each half, with the bottom of the kidney right around the bottom of your rib cage. Some inches above that (ladies can use the back of their bras as a locator) sits an adrenal gland, topping the kidney like a little beanie.

The adrenals handle our everyday energy needs, plus our fight-or-flight response in stressful situations. Healthy adrenals don't even let you know they're on the job; they just quietly go about their complicated business. Unfortunately, these babies own an uncanny ability to get into trouble.

If heavy stress goes on and on, they can conk out in adrenal fatigue, which is fixable if you take care of business. The first advice you'll hear is to get rid of your stress, which may or may not be possible. Here's some advice you generally won't hear: Get to bed by 10 pm every night and get good nutrition.

Any form of sugar stomps on the adrenals, so get rid of sugar–even though you probably crave it. Instead of sweets, eat fatty protein. (Saturated fat is the endocrine system's friend. Brain, too.) Then add a good program of vitamins and minerals to your daily routine so your adrenals have something to work with.

Adrenals can go down in flames trying to help a bum thyroid. And treating the thyroid without first meeting the needs of your adrenals do them in, too.

http://BetteDowdell.com

A damaged hypothalamus can cause adrenal problems, as can a whacked out pituitary. And things in the environment. And so forth.

Symptoms of adrenal problems are a lot like those of the thyroid–constant fatigue, brain fog, hair loss, sleep problems, etc. Symptoms specific to the adrenals include an itchy back, a patchy loss of leg hair and difficulty in word recall, especially names.

Another charmer is constant turmoil in your gastrointestinal system.

Then there's everybody's favorite symptom: the poochy belly. Even if you lose weight (if you can), it's still there.

Then there's your hair color. You're a long way down the road to adrenal failure when your hair, besides having a part as wide as a country lane, turns dark. Actually changes color. I went from light brown with a natural wave to poker-straight, mousy dark brown hair. All of a sudden, dark roots appeared.

Plus there's the fun of reacting to sudden noises by jumping out of your skin.

We're not talking about a picnic here.

Most doctors use blood tests to check the adrenals, which makes no sense at all. First off, it measures adrenal levels in the blood, not in the tissues where the action happens. Second, accurate tests of adrenal function span many hours. A one-shot blood test doesn't do the job–especially since it tests the wrong thing.

Doctors who test properly use either a saliva test or a 24-hour urine test.

Regardless of which test you get, meds may not be the way to go. I got my best results–well, actually, my only positive results–from the things I did for myself.

http://BetteDowdell.com

The Sugar-Balancing Pancreas

The **pancreas** is below our stomach, front and center, near the bottom of the rib cage. It may be the busiest twelve inches going.

The hormone-producing, endocrine part of the pancreas emits its hormones into the blood stream where they meet up with receptors that allow them to do what they were born to do: Control blood sugar.

The pancreas produces two hormones, insulin and glucagon, to handle our sugar levels. To lower blood sugar, it shoots out insulin. To raise blood sugar, it pumps glucagon.

Like the rest of the endocrine system, the pancreas works in bits and bursts, not a steady flow of hormones. So your body works 24/7, shooting out insulin now, glucagon then, to keep your blood sugar in balance–a ballet of exquisitely intricate choreography.

We can control some things that take the pancreas down: excessive or binge drinking for one–which may be why liver problems often accompany diabetes. High fructose corn syrup for another; that's huge. Beer seems to be a problem, but not dry wines. Vitamin and mineral deficiencies are huge, too.

A low/no fat diet, like that promoted by diabetes associations, creates an endocrine catastrophe. Saturated fat promotes endocrine health and also helps maintain good blood sugar levels. Why wouldn't we want to get some of that good stuff?

Other fats, including liquid vegetable oils and their partially-hydrogenated brethren, aka transfats, create inflammation, which in turn creates diabetes–among many other diseases.

Too little insulin leads to Type 1 diabetes. In Type 2 diabetes, you have enough insulin, but your body doesn't want anything to do with it, so it's like you don't have enough. Hypoglycemia, on the other hand, has you drowning in insulin, which, since fainting's pretty common in hypoglycemia, can leave you in a heap on the floor.

If you eat something sweet, say a doughnut or a piece of cake, on an empty stomach, checking how you feel an hour later can give you a good clue. If you're wired, perspiring and light-headed, you really need to be tested for diabetes. If, on the other hand, you feel like a truck hit you, and all you want to do is sleep–which you may do wherever you are or whatever time it is–you may be dealing with hypoglycemia.

Now, you don't want to purposefully create problems for yourself, but if you find yourself in difficulty, check back to what you ate/drank an hour before and see if there's a connection.

Write this on a rock: If you have diabetes, you also have significant nutritional deficiencies. Always. Which is just one reason I jump up and down about nutrition all the time.

http://BetteDowdell.com

The Endangered Gonads

The gonads, our **testes** and **ovaries**, play a huge role in how the endocrine system works. And we seem to be doing everything we can to put them on the disabled list. We need to talk about this.

Everybody has–and needs–estrogen, progesterone and testosterone. Now, obviously men and women, boys and girls have different levels of these hormones. But who knows how long that's going to last? Testosterone levels have fallen way, way down over the last forty years or so. Estrogen levels, meanwhile, have skyrocketed.

Our bodies, though, prefer the original plan and really put up a stink about what's happening. Which makes the rest of the endocrine system unhappy like you wouldn't believe.

Women get to deal with PMS, endometriosis and a difficult menopause. Little boys suffer through lifelong low testosterone and fertility problems. Little girls make a precocious leap for puberty–at which point, they start with the PMS, difficult periods, etc. Men, not to be left out, start converting testosterone into estrogen, develop breasts–aka moobs–and lose their libido. And everybody heads for the cancer line: Males for prostate cancer and women for cancers of one or more of the female organs, particularly the breast.

Why in the world are we doing this to ourselves? And how?

http://BetteDowdell.com

As I said before, endocrine glands emit hormones as needed. The hormones roam about until they find a receptor that fits, a kind of lock and key arrangement. Locking in releases the hormone's power and glory.

But if a pretender reaches the receptor before the real hormone comes along, it locks up the receptor, taking it out of play. The real hormone has no place to go. Some hormones simply wash out, but not estrogen. It gets seriously unhappy and starts making trouble. Big trouble.

And it happens every day, but we don't even realize we're surrounded by enemies. We live in a dangerous world of bogus, pretender estrogen.

Here's a pretender-estrogen enemies list

- Soy is enemy #1. It's everywhere, in most of our food and some of our lotions and potions. It strips away our minerals, depresses the thyroid gland and pours a boatload of bogus estrogen into us. Food manufacturers try to cover it up by using a variety of names. Just know it's in all processed foods–fast food, chain restaurant food, any meal you buy in a box or the grocery store freezer.

- Flax is soy's equally ugly cousin.

- Phthalate, the additive that makes plastic soft and pliable–as in a baby's teething ring, baby bottles and medical tubing–and a world of other stuff. The FDA started talking about the problem in 1980; so far, though, nothing.

- Plastic containers with a recycle code (in a triangle, usually on the bottom) of 1, 3 or 7.

- Parabens, chemicals added to our lotions and potions to extend shelf life. If you see an ingredient that ends in paraben (sometimes you'll see as many as six), put the product back on the shelf and walk away. And don't you dare put that stuff on children!

- Most food cans get lined with BPA, a synthetic estrogen. It prevents food/can chemical reactions, but seeps into the food. And computers contain BPA, too. Lots of things. And nobody has to tell you it's there.

- Birth control pills, both those taken on purpose and the second-hand ingredients that enter our homes via the municipal water supply. HRT, too.

- And on, and on.

If enough of us get a clue and start making noise–if only with our spending choices–manufacturers will change the way they do things. In the meantime, protecting our health from bogus estrogen takes some attention and effort.

Or you can just go along and hope for the best. After all, not all smokers get lung cancer, and not all people who play footsy with estrogen get breast or prostate cancer. How lucky do you feel?

Your Protector: The Thymus

Our thymus gland lies behind our breast bone. It's all about our immune system.

Thymus cells, T-cells, help our bodies recognize and destroy marauding bacteria, viruses and whatever else tries to attack us. They also guard against abnormal cell growth, as in cancer, and any foreign tissues that gets into our bodies.

A wobbly thymus leads us down a bad path that can end in any one of the autoimmune diseases; which disease shows up depends on where the weakest link in our body is.

Your immune system can't be 'too strong.' Out of whack, yes. Too powerful, no.

But the medicines given for autoimmune diseases are all based on the theory that your immune system is too strong. Which is probably why they don't work.

For years, we were told that the thymus gland atrophies and turns into fat as we age. However, twenty years ago or so, researchers proved that theory wrong. A healthy thymus remains robust throughout life.

Cadavers, the source of the shrunken thymus theory, do have tiny thymus glands. Not, however, because the gland atrophied over the years, but because a thymus under attack from severe illness, such as a terminal illness, or enormous stress gets depleted from fighting the battle at hand. It shrivels up to next to nothing in less than 24 hours. It's not dead; it just needs some rest and TLC.

So, how do we keep our thymus gland properly plumped up? Vitamins, minerals, exercise and the avoidance of unhealthy foods and pollutants.

While this is not exactly rocket science, it doesn't seem to be understood in all circles. Doctors tell patients, especially those fight cancer, heart disease, diabetes–you know, the biggies–to avoid vitamins and minerals because they might interfere with proper treatment. So just when the thymus needs all the support it can get, we put it on a starvation diet. Swell. Especially since vitamins and minerals, as it turns out, help and don't cause any problems.

And in your diet, add the good and avoid the bad. Again, not rocket science.

Finally, people near death, with no hope of recovery, can sometimes be returned to excellent health with an injection of thymus extract. In 1967 a doctor/researcher announced that this practice, and its miraculous results, would become standard practice within five or ten years. Nothing yet, though.

The Balancing Parathyroids

Close by the thyroid lie four similarly named, but unrelated, endocrine glands, the parathyroids. These tiny glands, each the size of a grain of rice, control our calcium balance.

Calcium provides electrical energy to our muscles and nerves.

When our blood calcium level runs low, the parathyroid hormones release calcium from our bones, prevent its loss in our urine and enhance calcium absorption in our intestines to build—to get it back up where it belongs.

It may seem that the easy way to fix the problem is to take calcium, but that can actually make things worse.

Here's how: Calcium hits the skids when magnesium is scarce—as it usually is in today's world. Our bodies balance calcium and magnesium 24/7; if magnesium levels are low, we dump calcium until it reaches magnesium's level—even if we end up without enough of either.

If we take calcium, but don't balance it out with magnesium, it just means there's more calcium to dump. And a tsunami of calcium on its way out may go places it shouldn't—such as arteries, heart valves and parathyroids.

High calcium causes our parathyroids to falter, causing fatigue, osteoporosis, kidney stones, heartburn, bone pain, heart palpitations, depression, headaches, an increased risk of breast or

http://BetteDowdell.com

prostate cancer, sleep difficulties and general grumpiness. Or you may be symptom-free and discover the problem coincidentally.

Or we may have a parathyroid tumor; typically on only one parathyroid gland.

And kidney disease makes life hard on the parathyroids.

In many, if not most, parathyroid problems, the glands ended up as collateral damage in removal of the thyroid gland. This shouldn't happen, but it does. Sometimes they even whack all four. Which is another reason to try natural ways to fix hyperthyroidism before even thinking about slicing and dicing.

http://BetteDowdell.com

The Mysterious Pineal

Deep in your brain, in a made-to-fit alcove, sits the **pineal** (PIN ee uhl) gland, the subject of much conjecture and not so much research.

Mystics call the pineal "The Third Eye" and tie it to extrasensory experiences. And they write more about it than scientists.

But I found some good science, so lets talk about that.

The pineal produces melatonin to run our body-clock through our 24-hour circadian cycles and seasonal adjustments. One word about our internal clock: A strong pineal gland hates changes in its routine, and it doesn't change its routine to fit your schedule.

This explains jet lag problems. Who gave you permission to get off schedule? Actually, jet lag says your pineal gland's ready to rumble. On the other hand, if you can change your schedule any which way without getting jet lag, your pineal's in trouble.

And taking melatonin is probably not the answer. While it may seem like an easy, logical response to a problem, it's way more complicated than popping a pill.

It's not dangerous to take melatonin, but it usually doesn't work right. Either nothing happens or it works too well, turning you into a zombie–which makes getting out of bed in the morning a real trick. But once you leave zombie-land, you're good to go.

What does the pineal in? First, as you might guess, would be problems anywhere else in the endocrine system. Especially if the problem is with the adrenals or the thymus.

Second, toxins do bad things to the pineal. For instance, fluoride.

The pineal and thyroid both take a huge hit from fluoride, with the pineal probably getting the worst of the deal. It absorbs more fluoride than other body parts, and turns into rock.

Well, rocks can't make hormones, so there goes melatonin. Bummer! Both the adrenals and thymus need melatonin and swoon when they can't get it.

We need to rethink fluoride. It's a hazardous, poisonous material that requires handlers to wear haz-mat outfits–complete with masks. If they dump fluoride into a river, they go to jail. If they dump it into our water supply, they get paid. What's that about?

Especially since all the talk about doing good things for our teeth is bogus. It does nothing good for our teeth, and it causes all sorts of problems for the rest of our bodies. Bottom line, we're paying to be poisoned.

http://BetteDowdell.com

A Courtesy From Your Fat Cells: Leptin

Leptin's a new kid on the block. Well, it's an old thing because it's been around, doing its thing, forever. But who knew?

Leptin comes from our body fat. Yikes! While our blubber isn't actually a gland, what it does and how it does it (emitter/receptor) makes it part of the endocrine family.

Anyway, our white fat–our blubber, as opposed to brown fat, which is good fat–is chock-a-block full of endocrine hormones–with new ones being discovered, it seems, almost daily. Chief among these hormones is leptin, which tells us when to stop eating, and grehlin, which encourages us to chow down. When both work well, we remain slim and trim.

But the food industry and our lack of knowledge are conspiring against leptin, which is very bad news.

Case in point: high fructose corn syrup. Our bodies don't know how to handle it, so it marches in and starts breaking the furniture.

Whenever we eat or drink something that confuses our bodies, such as HFCS, it gets dumped into our liver for clean-up. Well, even the liver doesn't know what to do with HFCS, so it hits like a toxic bomb.

http://BetteDowdell.com

And what does this have to do with leptin? Leptin takes one look at HFCS and says, "Who Dat?," and it's not talking football.

Leptin can't handle HFCS, so it ignores it. Which means leptin never signals the brain to stop eating/drinking because you've had enough. Can you say "obesity epidemic?" And can you say "osteoporosis?"

How about "diabetes?" As it turns out, insulin and leptin are inseparable, and they tend to get in trouble together.

HFCS raises uric acid levels, too, moving you to the agony of gout. And to kidney damage. That stuff is murder!

Need more unhappy news? Okay. Remember the all-for-one, one-for-all nature of the endocrine system? Whenever a part of the endocrine system, leptin for instance, takes a hit, all the other endocrine glands try to make things right, often with the unfortunate result of taking down an innocent gland or two.

My obvious advice? Get HFCS out of your life. Don't include even a little bit in what you eat or drink. It's everywhere, so this will involve reading lots of labels, but your health will thank you.

Can These Bones Walk?

If we think of bones at all, we think of them kind of like sticks–firm, solid, inert. But bones get testy when you accuse them of being inert; bones are busy, busy, busy.

Like every other cell in our bodies, old bone cells are constantly replaced by new bone cells.

Osteoblasts bring in new bone cells. Osteoclasts cart away the dead bone cells.

The endocrine hormone osteocalcin, which is created by our bones, keeps the osteoblasts in business, building away.

And here's where good thyroid health comes in. Osteocalcin needs the calcitonin from our thyroid hormone to accomplish what it needs to accomplish.

Question: Does the use of Synthroid, which contains no calcitonin, to treat hypothyroid problems play a role in the huge–and growing–increase in osteoporosis problems? Yes, but nobody's checking.

It's bad enough that Synthroid doesn't help thyroid problems, which leads to all sorts of dread disease. Setting patients up for osteoporosis, too, is well beyond reasonable limits.

http://BetteDowdell.com

Research tells us osteocalcin does a whole lot more than build bones. It plays a role in controlling sugar levels, preventing obesity and providing energy.

Another question: Does osteocalcin need calcitonin to do its insulin work as well as its bone work? Again, nobody's checking yet, but then, the discovery that our bones are part of our endocrine system is too new to have many answers. But somebody needs to check this out; millions of patients may be in jeopardy.

One thing researchers know–but aren't talking about–is osteoporosis drugs damage our bones. These drugs prevent the osteoclasts from carting away the dead bone cells, so you end up with bones full of dead cells. Thick and good-looking in an x-ray, they're actually weak, brittle and easily broken. Just say "no."

Digestion

Now the poobahs think perhaps they should designate our digestion as a endocrine function. Strangely enough, this makes a lot of sense.

If your digestion insists on doing the fandango all the time, you almost surely have endocrine problems.

Adrenal problems, for instance, make hash of the small intestine. Add that to the low stomach acid that comes with thyroid problems, and your digestion's down for the count.

You may get a diagnosis of leaky gut syndrome, irritable bowel disease, even Crohn's Disease, but start working on making life easier for your endocrine system. That's much more likely to be where the problem–and the solution–starts.

I found this out the hard way. After a gastroenterologist made a really bad situation worse, I realized it was up to me, once again, and started to research.

While I knew my endocrine system didn't walk in victory, I had never read about its tight connection to the small intestine. Well, as it turns out, they are inseparable.

http://BetteDowdell.com

A lot of what the endocrine system does, it does in the small intestine. Besides the digestion that happens there, hormone emitters and receptors are everywhere.

We know, for instance, that the thyroid gland emits thyroid hormone, but so does the small intestine. How's that for a news bulletin?

So if your small intestine gets out of sorts, thyroid function goes down. Perhaps you wondered why you felt so tired.

Yeah, making digestion part of the endo system makes sense.

And there's talk about adding the brain to the endocrine system.

Why not? After all, estrogen plays a role in how our brains work.

Here's the bottom line: When it comes to our health, everything affects everything.

Health problems don't come in small, separate-from-everything-else packages. They may appear to at times, though, since the cause of a problem often lies hidden and far away from the seemingly unrelated result.

One thing for sure, you always find the endocrine system in the middle of every health hiccup. Perhaps the problem starts there. Or perhaps the endo system ends up as a victim. Or maybe it's a Good Samaritan just trying to help out.

The absolute fact is the better care you take of your endocrine system, the less likely that you will have to deal with illness.

http://BetteDowdell.com

Some Typical Endocrine Symptoms

Endocrine problems present an amazing variety of overlapping symptoms–hundreds and hundreds of them. And since endocrine glands always get into each other's business, untangling everything can be daunting.

It's not for nothing that doctors prefer to use blood tests. They get an answer–whether right or, more likely, wrong–in a trice.

We need at least a little help to figure things out. So here are a few of the typical symptoms related to endocrine glands gone astray.

Symptoms found in most endocrine problems:
- Fatigue like you wouldn't believe
- Loss of scalp hair
- Brain fog
- Lack of concentration
- Weight problems
- Loss of libido

Symptoms of an underactive pituitary:
- Loss of underarm hair
- Loss of pubic hair
- Answer phone in sleep
- Thyroid problems
- Adrenal problems
- Hypoglycemia
- Lack of growth hormone

http://BetteDowdell.com

- Subdued emotions

Symptoms of an overactive pituitary:
Almost always caused by a tumor. Symptoms depend on where the tumor is.
- A prolactin tumor generates milk discharge
- An adrenal tumor causes Cushing's Disease
- A growth hormone tumor causes giantism
- A thyroid tumor causes hyperthyroidism

Hypothyroid symptoms:
- Low blood pressure
- Constipation
- High cholesterol
- Craving for fat
- Sluggish emotional response
- Puffy eyes
- Feelings of depression
- Frequently feels cold
- Lose outer part of eyebrows
- Inside of ears itch
- Long, heavy, painful menstrual periods
- Muscle, joint pains
- Weight gain

Hyperthyroid symptoms:
- Racing heart, rapid pulse
- Eye pain
- Nervousness
- Weight loss
- High blood pressure
- Can't handle heat
- Increased activity

Symptoms of adrenal exhaustion
- Low blood pressure
- Low blood sugar

- Fast, irritable bowels
- Low cholesterol
- Crave salt
- Digestion usually in an uproar
- Emotional variability
- Sunken eyes with dark circles
- Hot one minute, cold the next
- Patchy hair loss on lower legs
- Heart valve problems
- Itchy back
- Vitiligo
- Headaches

Symptoms of overactive adrenals:
- Elevated blood sugar
- "Moon" face (also with hypothyroid)
- Red face and neck
- Swollen legs and/or feet
- Irritability

Symptoms of a broken-down thymus:
- Every germ and/or virus does you in
- Autoimmune diseases
- Digestive problems

Symptoms of too much (usually bogus) estrogen:
- Menstrual problems–all of 'em
- Endometriosis
- Menopause hits like a tornado
- Low testosterone levels
- Men convert testosterone to estrogen
- Men grow breasts
- Enlarged prostate
- Breast/Prostate cancer

Symptoms of a damaged hypothalamus:
- Anorexia, bulimia, obesity

http://BetteDowdell.com

- Erratic body temperature
- Never get hungry

Symptoms of high blood sugar - diabetes:
- Constant, excessive thirst
- Frequent infections
- Wounds heal slowly
- Irritability

Symptoms of low blood sugar - hypoglycemia:
- Trouble staying awake
- Feel shaky and anxious
- Heart palpitations
- Fainting

http://BetteDowdell.com

The Problem With Doctors

Endocrine patients know one thing for certain: Getting good medical care requires the patience of Job and persistence of a bill collector.

Knowing what's going on "behind the scenes," as it were, helps us determine whether or not to stay with a doctor and, if we stay, how to get the best results.

Why is it so hard?

First, let's recognize that some doctors don't care–either about you or about your problems. They read a book, and they're going to go by that book. If what they read in the book doesn't fix your so-called problem, then you're a difficult patient who refuses to conform–to the book.

You'd think after even a few years of one non-conforming patient after another, they'd catch a clue that perhaps the book has it wrong, but no. They know what they know, and that's that.

No imagination. No curiosity. Just an insistence on the rubber-stamp medicine of the book.

Fortunately, this description doesn't represent the majority of doctors, although endocrinologists seem to be over-represented in this unhappy gathering.

As a patient, you have two choices: Stay, with the continuing misery that staying entails, or leave to seek another doctor. Thinking anything you say or do will change the doctor's attitude is about the same as believing it's possible to shape concrete after it's already set.

And know this: When a doctor takes a condescending, my-way-or-the-highway approach, it's not about you. It's all about the doctor.

But avoiding disinterested doctors isn't the whole story.

Standard of Care

Arizona, where I live, is a standard-of-care state–as are many others, although that's kind of a secret that you have to discover on your own.

Let me describe in a nutshell what this means: Patients get one-size-fits-all treatment, whether it works or not.

Big Pharma and Big Insurance muscle their way onto State Medical Boards. Once there, they use that significant power to shut down real medicine. If healing happens, it's not because of them.

The Board sets standards for each medical condition, which sounds hopeful. However, the standards are intended to minimize costs and guarantee legal protection to doctors no matter what happens to patients.

For instance, the standard of care for thyroid is the TSH test, ignoring the fact this test is perhaps the premier example of unreliability, and standard treatment is Synthroid or a generic equivalent. Synthroid doesn't work for the vast majority of us. That's bad enough, but it causes an allergic reaction in lots of folks. So the TSH test is bogus, the only medicine allowed doesn't help and may harm, your hair continues to fall out, your brain continues to be lost in a pea-soup fog and life loses its joy. But the standard of care has been met.

And standard-of-care State Medical Boards don't approve of the adrenal saliva test, although it's accurate while their preferred bloods tests are pointless. So adrenal problems remain unaddressed and untreated, wreaking all sorts of health havoc. If your adrenals are suffering, so are you–in spades.

And it's not just about endocrine problems. State Boards decree normal cholesterol levels are too high and insist doctors prescribe statin drugs to lower them–although cholesterol has nothing to do with heart disease and statins are a disaster, with serious side effect upon serious side effect.

Research says statins save well less than one life per twenty years of male (statins don't work at all for women) patient suffering and expense, a major failure. Even so, any diagnosis of heart problems includes a prescription for a statin drug, even if you don't have high cholesterol–which describes more than half of heart patients.

And on and on. Standard-of-care means inferior care.

And your doctor can't do anything different from standard-of-care without risking his/her medical license. A doctor I admire said she fears the State Medical Board above everything.

Want more? If you refuse to do as you're told, the doctor's supposed to dismiss you as a patient.

Arizona has a doctor shortage, at least in part because doctors are leaving. They want to practice medicine in a state that still allows them to use their knowledge and skills to treat patients. Those states are few and far between.

Because of the Arizona State Medical Board, I've lost some doctors, and I've made others crazy by my unwillingness to ride with the tide. I recognize the doctor's dilemma, but, golly gee whiz, I'm not about to live half a life.

Fortunately, my years of study give me a huge edge in self-care. So I try to break doctors in with the idea of being a coach. I'll study, I'll experiment on myself and I'll tell them all about it if–and I have to be really diplomatic here–they'll cough up a prescription for natural, desiccated thyroid.

This asks a lot of doctors. Although desiccated thyroid has proved its worth again and again–for more than a century now–standard-of-care disapproves of it. Strongly. Why? As usual, follow the money.

So, if your doctor shows little flexibility or initiative, it may be that he's dying inside, but he has a family and many thousands of dollars in student loans, so he can't risk his license. Military doctors lose everything by prescribing a decent thyroid medication.

Given this reality, we have to learn how our bodies work and what they need to live in health. We can take care of most of what we need to do. It's great to have a doctor to guide us along, but even then, what we do for ourselves will improve the outcome.

Especially since doctors don't study nutrition in medical school and know about as much about it as, say, a journalist who also hasn't studied it.

Standard of care never, ever includes nutrition.

Endocrine Enemies

• A low-fat diet •
• A low-protein diet •
• Polyunsaturated vegetable oils •
• Hydrogenated/partially hydrogenated fats or oils •
• Aspartame •
• MSG (monosodium glutamate) •
• Soy •
• Flax •
• High fructose corn syrup •
• Bromine (in bread, Mountain Dew, etc.) •
• Meat from factory farms (meat sold at the grocery stores) •
• Milk from factory farms (milk sold at grocery stores) •

• Fluoride •
• Chlorine •

• Birth control pills •
• Hormone replacement therapy •
• Fluoride-containing antibiotics •
• Fluoride-containing antidepressants •
• Statin drugs •

Resources

- Subscribe to my free, weekly health e-zine:
  http://TooPoopedToParticipate.com

Your immediate prize is a list of the most common symptoms I talk about so you can see if they're part of your deal.

And you'll get a health article each Tuesday morning to keep you up-to-date on where research is going–both in what to do and what not to do.

This is the kind of help you need to feel better.

I'm all about providing life-enhancing information to improve your health. I got myself out of the ditch; you can, too.

And you can unsubscribe any time.

What's not to love?

- Get my e-book on the basic vitamins and minerals that everybody needs, *Pep for the Pooped: Discovering the vitamins and minerals your body is starving for.*

  http://PepForThePooped.com

http://BetteDowdell.com

- Cut to the chase and join the *Moving to Health* Membership program.

This low-cost program provides a step-by-step education about understanding how your body works, what you can do to help it along–and, finally, to become your own, best health advocate.

Members receive new information every week for a year, including links to quality vitamins et al. I receive no money for these recommendations; they're all about you.

Each week builds on what you've already learned, and you'll be able to make health improvements each step of the way.

And I cover pretty much everything from autism to weight loss.

There's nothing else like *Moving to Health* anywhere.

Research proves the endocrine system is smack dab in the middle of health–but few people, including doctors, seem to understand this.

Happily, most people will do whatever it takes to get healthy–once they know what to do–which is where *Moving to Health* comes in.

Since everybody's different (You can say that again!), I give you the information you need to diagnose your own problems so you can start making improvements.

You're the only one who knows how you feel, so you're the best person to make your diagnosis.

I'll admit it takes effort. But can you tell me something wonderful that doesn't?

http://BetteDowdell.com

I started my health recovery lower than a snake's belly, with hardly enough energy to get through a day. But those days are gone forever, and life is good.

The truth is, our bodies work self-healing magic when they get the support they need.

Read the details at http://MovingToHealth.com

- Subscribe to both *Too Pooped to Participate* and *Moving to Health*. They complement each other, so you won't be duplicating.

http://TooPoopedToParticipate.com
http://MovingToHealth.com

KNOWLEDGE IS POWER!

http://BetteDowdell.com

Index

Absorption. 53
Acid. 34, 39, 58, 61
Adrenals. 3, 5, 10, 17, 19, 23, 24, 26, 28, 43, 44, 55, 56, 65, 69
Aging. 5, 27, 33
Antibiotics. 40, 71
Antibodies. 34, 35
Antibody. 35
Antidepressants. 71
Anxiety. 31
Arthritis. 20
Autism. 73
Autoimmune. 9, 20, 21, 35, 51, 65
Blood. 12, 17, 19, 31, 33-37, 44, 45, 53, 63-66
Blood pressure. 64
Bones. 3, 5, 10, 17, 18, 24, 34, 53, 59, 60
Brain. 5, 6, 9, 10, 12, 15, 16, 19, 21, 23, 31, 39, 43, 44, 55, 57,
62, 63, 68
Breast cancer. 13
Calcitonin. 34, 37, 59
Calcium. 16, 53
Cancer. 12, 13, 17, 47, 49, 51-53, 65
Children. 27, 48
Cholesterol. 37, 39, 64, 69
Concentration. 63
Constipation. 64
Dementia. 23
Depression. 31, 53, 64
Diabetes. 45, 46, 65
Digestion. 3, 61, 62, 64
Diuretic. 26
Endometriosis. 12, 47, 65
Estrogen. 10, 12, 13, 17, 21, 40, 47-49, 62, 65
Estrogen dominance. 12, 17
Exercise. 52
Fat. 3, 17, 18, 24, 40, 43, 45, 51, 57, 64, 71
Fatigue. 16, 19, 31, 43, 44, 53, 63
Fibromyalgia. 32
Fluoride. 12, 56, 71
Food sensitivities. 35
Gall bladder. 40
GERD. 39

Glutamate..21, 71
Gout. 58
Grass-fed... 40
Growth hormone............................. 26, 27, 63, 64
Hair loss. 16, 31, 44, 65
Headaches. 53, 65
Heart. 31, 32, 36, 52, 53, 64-66, 69
Heart valve... 65
Heartburn.. 53
High blood pressure.................................... 64
Hormones.................. 10-12, 18, 19, 24, 26, 27, 40, 45, 47, 48, 53, 56,
                                                       57
Hypoglycemia............................... 17, 46, 63, 66
Hypothalamus. 3, 5, 10, 15, 19-23, 25-27, 33, 43, 65
Hypothyroid. 32, 35, 36, 38, 59, 64, 65
Immune................................... 16, 32, 51
Immune system................................... 16, 51
Infections. 40, 65
Inflammation. 45
Insulin. 45, 46, 58, 59
Intestines. 53
Iodine................................... 12, 34, 38
Irritability. 65, 66
Kidney.............................. 43, 53, 54, 58
Kidney stones.................................... 53
Kidneys...16, 40
Leptin.............................3, 10, 18, 19, 57, 58
Libido................................... 12, 47, 63
Liver................................... 40, 45, 57
Low blood pressure. 64
Low stomach acid. 39, 61
Low-fat diet. 71
Low-protein diet. 71
Magnesium. 53
Melatonin.................................. 16, 55, 56
Menopause................................... 12, 47, 65
Monosodium glutamate. 71
MSG.................................... 20, 21, 71
Muscles................................... 53
Nerves.................................... 53
Neuropathy.................................... 22
Nutrition................................. 6, 20, 35, 43, 46, 70
Obesity. 59, 65
Oxytocin. 26

Pain..53, 64
Palpitations.. 31, 53, 66
Pancreas.................................... 3, 5, 10, 17, 19, 24, 28, 45
Parathyroids............................... 3, 5, 10, 16, 19, 24, 38, 53, 54
Parkinson's. 6, 23
pH..37, 68
Pineal.. 3, 5, 10, 16, 19, 24, 55, 56
Pituitary........................ 3, 5, 6, 10, 15, 16, 19, 23-28, 32, 33, 43, 63
Progesterone.. 17, 40, 47
Prolactin.. 63
Prostate.. 12, 47, 49, 53, 65
Prostate cancer. 12, 47, 49, 53, 65
Protein.. 40, 43, 71
Receptor.. 11, 12, 17, 18, 47, 57
Receptors... 10-12, 45, 61
REM. 51, 57, 68
Salt. 26, 64
Saturated fat. 40, 43, 45
Skin...25, 44
Small intestine. 61
Statin drugs... 39, 69, 71
Statins..39, 69
Stomach. 17, 39, 45, 46, 61
Symptoms. 3, 27, 31, 32, 34, 35, 38, 39, 44, 63-66, 72
Temperature...19, 65
Testosterone.. 12, 13, 17, 40, 47, 65
Thymus..................... 3, 5, 10, 16, 19, 21, 24, 51, 52, 55, 56, 65
Thyroid................ 3, 10, 12, 15-17, 21, 23-28, 31-40, 43, 48, 53, 54, 56,
                                        59, 61, 63, 64, 68, 70
Toxins. 56
Type 2 diabetes. 46
Tyrosine. 34
Urine. 12, 44, 53
Vaccines. 21
Vasopressin.. 26
Vitamin A. 45
Weight.. 9, 31, 40, 44, 63, 64, 73
Weight gain. 64
Weight loss. 64, 73

http://BetteDowdell.com

What People Are Saying

Here's what a South Carolina reader says:
"God sent me to you and through all your research and hard work I have found healing from many years of suffering. I knew I wasn't depressed, "crazy" or truly debilitated --and I knew there was a root cause to my issues; you helped me find that cause."

-Allison Rooke

Here's a note of triumph from Florida:
I had Rheumatoid Arthritis, scoliosis, memory problems, nerve troubles, and menopausal symptoms that let me get only about 4 hours of sleep at night. I walked with a walker. I was at the end of my rope.

Bette, you have given me a new lease on life. When I began the MTH program, I was overwhelmed. I had problems concentrating, but the pain in my body gave me the incentive to press on. So I began reading over and over until I could comprehend enough to get me started. I had to unlearn all the things that I had been taught about healthy eating and exercising.

A year and a half later, I am on a full vitamin and mineral regimen. I did what you said and listened to my body (and still do). I can dance again, even jog some.

I got my memory back, and I was able to get my insurance agent's license.

I can't say enough about your program. It changed my life forever. Thank you, again and again.

Barbara Roman

And here's a word from British Columbia:
"Just wanted to let you know I am blown away by this course. I, as well as my family, was apprehensive, as we read scads of health info that leads to nowhere you might say. However, this is different. And I love your sense of humour. Thank you--take care."

Dianne Dawson

"Thank you for writing that brilliant book, *Pep for the Pooped*. It's the best info I have found making me able to do something for myself. Love to be told what to take and when. Really see some changes. Fantastic. I'm very grateful that you share all you know."

Hilde Rastad, Norway

Lisa from Down Under adds:
"Thank you. I am up to week 13. I am not where I need to be yet! But I'm not where I used to be !!!! Thank God. I order from your recommendations, and I have to say, I cannot believe the prices compared to Australia. Even including international postage, it's way cheaper than here! Downside is, I wait 4-6 weeks for them to arrive."

Lisa Cathro